Chapter 1: Introduction to Menstrual Health

Understanding the Menstrual Cycle

The menstrual cycle is a natural process that plays a crucial role in the reproductive health of individuals with a uterus. It typically lasts about 28 days, although cycles can range from 21 to 35 days. Understanding the different phases of the cycle can empower young adults to better manage their health and recognize what is normal for their bodies. The menstrual cycle is divided into four main phases: the menstrual phase, the follicular phase, ovulation, and the luteal phase.

The menstrual phase marks the beginning of the cycle and usually lasts between three to seven days. During this time, the lining of the uterus, which thickens in preparation for a potential pregnancy, sheds if fertilization has not occurred. This shedding results in menstruation, which includes bleeding from the vagina. It's important to note that the amount and duration of menstrual flow can vary widely among individuals. Some may experience heavy bleeding, while others may have lighter flows. Understanding these variations can help individuals identify what is typical for them and seek help if they notice significant changes.

Following the menstrual phase is the follicular phase, which lasts until ovulation. This phase begins on the first day of menstruation and is characterized by the development of follicles in the ovaries. Each follicle contains an egg, and during this phase, the hormone estrogen rises, stimulating the growth of the uterine lining in preparation for a potential pregnancy. This phase can vary in length but is generally around 14 days. The increase in estrogen can also lead to physical and emotional changes, such as increased energy levels and mood fluctuations.

Ovulation occurs approximately in the middle of the cycle, around day 14 in a typical 28-day cycle. During this phase, a mature egg is released from one of the ovaries and travels down the fallopian tube. This is the time when individuals are most fertile and can conceive if sperm is present. Ovulation is often accompanied by physical signs such as changes in cervical mucus, mild cramping, or increased libido. Understanding ovulation is essential for those who wish to conceive or avoid pregnancy, as recognizing the signs can help individuals better plan their reproductive choices.

The final phase of the menstrual cycle is the luteal phase, which lasts until the start of the next menstrual period. After ovulation, the ruptured follicle transforms into the corpus luteum, which produces progesterone. This hormone helps maintain the uterine lining, preparing it for a potential implantation of a fertilized egg. If fertilization does not occur, the levels of progesterone drop, leading to the breakdown of the uterine lining and the start of menstruation. This phase typically lasts about 14 days and can also bring about premenstrual symptoms such as bloating, mood swings, and breast tenderness. Recognizing these symptoms can help individuals manage their discomfort and better understand their cycles.

Importance of Menstrual Health

Menstrual health is a critical aspect of overall well-being that significantly impacts the lives of young adults. Understanding the menstrual cycle is not merely about managing monthly symptoms; it encompasses knowledge about reproductive health, emotional well-being, and lifestyle choices. A healthy menstrual cycle serves as an essential indicator of a person's overall health, reflecting hormonal balance, nutrition, and emotional state. Therefore, educating oneself about menstrual health can empower individuals to make informed decisions regarding their health and lifestyle.

One of the primary reasons menstrual health is important is its direct connection to reproductive health. Regular menstrual cycles indicate that the body is functioning properly, which is crucial for those who may wish to conceive in the future. Irregularities in the cycle can signal underlying health issues, such as hormonal imbalances or conditions like polycystic ovary syndrome (PCOS). By understanding what constitutes a normal cycle, young adults can recognize deviations that may warrant consultation with a healthcare provider, fostering proactive health management.

Moreover, menstrual health education plays a vital role in breaking down the stigma surrounding menstruation. Many young adults experience embarrassment or shame about their periods due to cultural taboos or lack of knowledge. By openly discussing menstrual health, individuals can create a more supportive environment where they feel comfortable sharing their experiences and seeking help when needed. This openness not only enhances personal well-being but also promotes a culture of acceptance and understanding among peers.

Emotional well-being is another essential factor linked to menstrual health. The hormonal fluctuations that occur during the menstrual cycle can significantly affect mood and mental health. Understanding these changes can help young adults develop coping strategies for mood swings, anxiety, or depression related to their cycles. Additionally, menstrual health education encourages individuals to prioritize self-care during their periods, fostering a holistic approach to mental and physical health.

Lastly, awareness of menstrual health can contribute to better lifestyle choices. Knowledge about nutrition, exercise, and stress management is crucial for maintaining a healthy cycle. For instance, a balanced diet rich in vitamins and minerals can alleviate symptoms like cramps and fatigue, while regular physical activity can enhance mood and reduce stress. By prioritizing menstrual health, young adults can cultivate habits that not only improve their cycles but also enhance their overall quality of life. This comprehensive understanding of menstrual health ultimately empowers individuals to take charge of their bodies and health, paving the way for a healthier future.

Chapter 2: Anatomy of the Female Reproductive System

Key Structures Involved

The menstrual cycle involves several key structures in the female reproductive system that work together to regulate the process. Understanding these structures is essential for grasping how menstruation occurs and how it affects overall health. The primary organs involved include the ovaries, fallopian tubes, uterus, and vagina, each playing a specific role in the cycle.

The ovaries are two almond-shaped glands located on either side of the uterus. They are responsible for producing eggs, or ova, and hormones such as estrogen and progesterone. Each month, during the menstrual cycle, one ovary releases an egg in a process called ovulation. This release typically occurs around the midpoint of the cycle, approximately two weeks before the onset of menstruation. The hormones produced by the ovaries help to prepare the body for a potential pregnancy.

Once the egg is released, it travels through the fallopian tubes, which connect the ovaries to the uterus. The fallopian tubes serve as the pathway for the egg, and they are also the site where fertilization can occur if sperm is present. If the egg is fertilized, it will continue its journey down the tube and implant itself into the lining of the uterus. If fertilization does not occur, the egg will disintegrate and the body will prepare for menstruation.

The uterus is a hollow, muscular organ where a fertilized egg can develop into a fetus. The inner lining of the uterus, known as the endometrium, thickens in preparation for a potential pregnancy each month. If the egg is not fertilized, the endometrial lining sheds, leading to menstruation. This process typically lasts between three to seven days and involves the expulsion of blood and tissue through the vagina.

The vagina serves as the canal through which menstrual fluid exits the body. It is also the passageway for sperm to enter the reproductive system during sexual intercourse. The health of the vagina is crucial for overall menstrual health, as it plays a role in maintaining an appropriate environment for the flora that help protect against infections. Recognizing and understanding these key structures not only helps in understanding the menstrual cycle but also empowers young adults to take charge of their reproductive health.

Hormones and Their Role

Hormones play a crucial role in the menstrual cycle, acting as chemical messengers that influence many bodily functions. Understanding these hormones is essential for recognizing how they affect physical and emotional health throughout the cycle. The primary hormones involved in regulating menstruation are estrogen, progesterone, luteinizing hormone (LH), and follicle-stimulating hormone (FSH). Each of these hormones has specific functions and interacts with the others to ensure the cycle progresses smoothly.

Estrogen is primarily produced by the ovaries and is responsible for the development of female secondary sexual characteristics. This hormone plays a significant role during the first half of the menstrual cycle, known as the follicular phase. As estrogen levels rise, they stimulate the thickening of the uterine lining in preparation for a potential pregnancy. Additionally, estrogen influences mood and energy levels, which can fluctuate throughout the month. Understanding how estrogen affects the body can help young adults manage their emotional well-being during different phases of the cycle.

Following ovulation, which occurs around the midpoint of the cycle, progesterone takes center stage. This hormone is crucial for maintaining the uterine lining, making it suitable for a fertilized egg to implant. If pregnancy does not occur, progesterone levels drop, leading to the shedding of the uterine lining, or menstruation.

Progesterone also affects mood and can lead to symptoms of premenstrual syndrome (PMS), such as irritability and fatigue. By recognizing the role of progesterone, individuals can better prepare for the emotional and physical changes that accompany their menstrual cycles.

Luteinizing hormone (LH) and follicle-stimulating hormone (FSH) are produced by the pituitary gland and play vital roles in regulating the menstrual cycle. FSH stimulates the growth of ovarian follicles, while LH triggers ovulation, signaling the release of an egg from the ovary. These hormones work in tandem to ensure the proper functioning of the reproductive system. Understanding their roles can empower young adults to grasp how their bodies work and the timing of ovulation within their cycles, which is essential for those considering pregnancy or tracking their fertility.

In summary, hormones are fundamental to understanding menstrual health. By learning about the roles of estrogen, progesterone, LH, and FSH, young adults can gain insight into their bodies and the changes they experience throughout the menstrual cycle. This knowledge not only helps in managing menstrual symptoms but also fosters a greater appreciation for the complexities of reproductive health. Embracing this understanding can lead to more informed decisions regarding health and wellness as individuals navigate their adolescent and young adult lives.

Chapter 3: The Menstrual Cycle Phases

The Follicular Phase

The follicular phase is the first part of the menstrual cycle, occurring after menstruation and lasting until ovulation. This phase generally lasts about 14 days, though it can vary depending on the individual. During this time, the body prepares for a potential pregnancy. The follicular phase begins on the first day of menstruation, which is considered day one of the cycle. As the cycle progresses, hormonal changes play a crucial role in regulating the development of follicles in the ovaries.

At the onset of the follicular phase, the levels of estrogen and progesterone are low. The pituitary gland, located at the base of the brain, releases follicle-stimulating hormone (FSH), which stimulates the ovaries to produce follicles. Each follicle contains an immature egg, and usually, one dominant follicle will emerge to continue maturing while the others undergo a process called atresia, where they stop growing. This selection process is vital for ensuring that the healthiest egg is available for potential fertilization.

As the dominant follicle develops, it begins to produce increasing amounts of estrogen. This rise in estrogen levels triggers a series of physiological changes in the body. The lining of the uterus thickens in preparation for a possible implantation of a fertilized egg, and the cervical mucus becomes more abundant and less viscous. These changes create a more favorable environment for sperm, should fertilization occur. The increase in estrogen also has an effect on mood and energy levels, often resulting in feelings of increased vitality and optimism.

The follicular phase can also be a time of heightened creativity and social interaction. Many individuals report feeling more outgoing and energized during this phase. Engaging in physical activities, pursuing hobbies, and connecting with friends can be particularly rewarding at this time. Understanding these fluctuations can help young adults harness their natural rhythms, allowing them to make the most of their energy and motivation.

As the follicular phase comes to a close, estrogen levels peak, leading to the triggering of luteinizing hormone (LH), which is responsible for initiating ovulation. This transition marks the end of the follicular phase and the beginning of the ovulatory phase. Recognizing the signs of the follicular phase can empower young adults to better understand their bodies, appreciate the complexities of their menstrual cycles, and make informed choices regarding their reproductive health.

Ovulation

Ovulation is a crucial part of the menstrual cycle, typically occurring around the midpoint of the cycle, which is approximately 14 days before the start of the next period. During this phase, an ovary releases a mature egg, which then travels down the fallopian tube. This process is influenced by hormones, particularly luteinizing hormone and follicle-stimulating hormone, which signal the ovaries to prepare for the release of an egg. Understanding ovulation is essential not only for those interested in conception but also for recognizing the natural rhythms of the body.

The menstrual cycle can be divided into several phases, with ovulation being the third phase, following the menstrual phase and the follicular phase. The follicular phase begins on the first day of menstruation and lasts until ovulation occurs. During this time, the body prepares for the possibility of pregnancy by thickening the uterine lining and maturing several follicles in the ovaries. Typically, one follicle becomes dominant and releases its egg during ovulation, while the others are reabsorbed by the body.

Timing your ovulation can be important for various reasons, including family planning. Many people track their cycles to identify their fertile window, which is the time when conception is most likely to occur. This window typically spans six days: five days leading up to ovulation and the day of ovulation itself. By using methods such as calendar tracking, observing changes in cervical mucus, or using ovulation predictor kits, individuals can gain insight into their ovulation patterns and improve their understanding of their reproductive health.

Additionally, ovulation can be accompanied by physical symptoms that vary from person to person. Some may experience a slight increase in basal body temperature, breast tenderness, or mild abdominal cramping known as mittelschmerz. These signs can serve as indicators of when ovulation is occurring. Being aware of these symptoms can help individuals better understand their cycles and recognize any irregularities that may warrant further attention from a healthcare provider.

It is also important to note that not everyone has a regular cycle, and factors such as stress, illness, and hormonal imbalances can affect ovulation. Conditions like polycystic ovary syndrome (PCOS) can lead to irregular ovulation or anovulation, where no egg is released at all. If you have concerns about your cycle or ovulation patterns, it is advisable to seek guidance from a healthcare professional. Understanding your body and its signaling can empower you to make informed decisions regarding your menstrual health and overall well-being.

The Luteal Phase

The luteal phase is a critical part of the menstrual cycle, occurring after ovulation and before the start of menstruation. This phase typically lasts around 10 to 14 days and is characterized by hormonal changes that prepare the body for a potential pregnancy. After an ovary releases an egg, the empty follicle transforms into the corpus luteum, which produces progesterone. This hormone plays a vital role in thickening the uterine lining, making it suitable for a fertilized egg to implant.

During the luteal phase, progesterone levels rise, while estrogen levels also fluctuate. These hormonal changes can lead to various physical and emotional symptoms. Many individuals may experience premenstrual syndrome (PMS), which can include mood swings, bloating, breast tenderness, and fatigue. Understanding these symptoms can help young adults differentiate between normal premenstrual changes and those that may require medical attention.

The luteal phase is not just about preparing for a possible pregnancy; it also plays a role in regulating the menstrual cycle. If the egg is not fertilized, the corpus luteum breaks down, leading to a decrease in progesterone levels. This drop triggers the shedding of the uterine lining, marking the beginning of menstruation. Knowing this process can empower young people to track their cycles and recognize their body's signals, promoting a healthier relationship with their menstrual health.

Lifestyle factors can also significantly influence the luteal phase. Diet, exercise, and stress levels can impact the severity of PMS symptoms and overall hormonal balance. Maintaining a well-balanced diet rich in vitamins and minerals, engaging in regular physical activity, and managing stress through relaxation techniques can help alleviate some of the discomfort associated with this phase. It's essential for young adults to develop healthy habits that support their menstrual health.

In conclusion, the luteal phase is an essential component of the menstrual cycle that involves intricate hormonal changes and physical symptoms. By understanding what occurs during this phase, young adults can better navigate their menstrual health and recognize the importance of self-care. Knowledge about the luteal phase empowers individuals to manage their symptoms and promotes a positive attitude towards their bodies and their cycles.

Menstruation

Menstruation is a natural biological process that typically begins during puberty, marking the start of a young woman's reproductive years. The average age for the onset of menstruation, also known as menarche, is around 12 years, but it can vary widely from 9 to 16 years. Menstruation occurs approximately every 28 days, although cycles can be shorter or longer. Understanding what happens during this cycle is essential for promoting menstrual health and addressing any concerns that may arise.

The menstrual cycle is divided into several phases: the menstrual phase, the follicular phase, ovulation, and the luteal phase. The menstrual phase begins with the shedding of the uterine lining, which results in menstrual bleeding. This phase typically lasts between three to seven days. Following this, the follicular phase begins, during which the body prepares for ovulation. Hormones released from the pituitary gland stimulate the ovaries to produce follicles, each containing an egg. This phase can vary in length, contributing to differences in cycle length among individuals.

Ovulation occurs approximately midway through the cycle, around day 14 in a typical 28-day cycle. During ovulation, a mature egg is released from the ovary and is available for fertilization. This is often the most fertile time in the cycle, and understanding this phase is crucial for those who may be considering pregnancy or practicing contraception. After ovulation, the luteal phase begins, during which the body prepares for a potential pregnancy. If fertilization does not occur, hormone levels drop, leading to the start of the next menstrual phase.

Menstrual symptoms can vary significantly among individuals. While some may experience mild symptoms such as cramping, bloating, or mood swings, others may face more severe issues like heavy bleeding or debilitating pain known as dysmenorrhea. It is important for young adults to recognize that these symptoms can be managed through various methods, including over-the-counter medications, lifestyle changes, and, in some cases, consultation with a healthcare professional for further guidance.

Understanding menstruation is not only about recognizing the physical changes that occur but also about fostering a positive attitude towards menstrual health. Open communication about menstrual issues can reduce stigma and encourage individuals to seek the help they need. Education about menstrual health empowers young adults to take charge of their bodies, understand their cycles, and make informed choices regarding their reproductive health.

Chapter 4: Common Menstrual Issues

PMS (Premenstrual Syndrome)

Premenstrual Syndrome (PMS) is a common condition that affects many individuals during the luteal phase of their menstrual cycle, typically one to two weeks before menstruation. It encompasses a range of physical and emotional symptoms that can vary significantly in severity and duration. While not all individuals experience PMS, those who do may notice symptoms such as mood swings, irritability, bloating, breast tenderness, fatigue, and changes in appetite. Understanding PMS is essential for young adults as it can impact daily life, relationships, and overall well-being.

The exact cause of PMS remains unclear, but researchers believe it is linked to hormonal fluctuations that occur throughout the menstrual cycle. During the luteal phase, levels of estrogen and progesterone rise and fall, which can affect neurotransmitters in the brain, particularly serotonin. This fluctuation may contribute to the emotional symptoms associated with PMS. Additionally, factors such as stress, lifestyle, and diet can exacerbate these symptoms, making it essential to consider a holistic approach to managing PMS.

Recognizing the symptoms of PMS is crucial for effective management. Young adults should take note of any patterns in their physical and emotional states during their cycle. Keeping a menstrual diary can help track symptoms, their intensity, and any potential triggers. This information can be beneficial when discussing PMS with healthcare providers, who can offer tailored advice and treatment options. Awareness of one's cycle not only empowers individuals to anticipate and address their symptoms but also fosters a greater understanding of their menstrual health.

There are various strategies for managing PMS symptoms, ranging from lifestyle modifications to medical interventions. Regular exercise, a balanced diet, and adequate sleep can significantly alleviate PMS symptoms for some individuals. Techniques such as yoga, mindfulness, and relaxation exercises can also help manage stress and improve emotional well-being. In some cases, over-the-counter medications like nonsteroidal anti-inflammatory drugs (NSAIDs) may provide relief from physical discomfort. For those with more severe symptoms, healthcare providers may recommend hormonal treatments or antidepressants as part of a comprehensive management plan.

Ultimately, PMS is a normal part of the menstrual cycle for many young adults, but it is crucial to approach it with education and self-care. By understanding the nature of PMS and recognizing its symptoms, individuals can take proactive steps to manage their health. Open discussions about menstrual health, whether with friends or healthcare professionals, can help break the stigma surrounding PMS and empower individuals to seek support when needed. Embracing menstrual health as an integral aspect of overall well-being is vital for fostering a positive relationship with one's body and cycle.

Irregular Periods

Irregular periods can be a common experience for many young adults, particularly during the first few years after menstruation begins. This irregularity can manifest in various ways, including varying cycle lengths, missed periods, or unexpected bleeding. Understanding what constitutes an irregular period is crucial for young adults as it can help demystify the changes their bodies are going through and empower them to take charge of their menstrual health.

Several factors can contribute to irregular periods. Hormonal fluctuations, stress, significant weight changes, and underlying health conditions can all play a role. For instance, the body produces hormones that regulate the menstrual cycle, and any imbalance in these hormones can lead to irregularities. Stress, both physical and emotional, can impact hormone levels, resulting in skipped or delayed periods. Similarly, excessive exercise or drastic changes in diet can affect menstrual regularity as the body adjusts to new routines.

It is important to note that occasional irregularities are generally not a cause for concern, especially during the initial years of menstruation. The body often takes time to establish a regular cycle, and fluctuations are normal as the reproductive system matures. However, if irregular periods persist or are accompanied by other concerning symptoms, such as severe pain, significant mood changes, or unusual discharge, it may be a sign to seek medical advice. Consulting a healthcare provider can help identify any underlying issues and provide guidance on managing menstrual health.

Tracking menstrual cycles can be an effective way for young adults to monitor their periods and identify patterns. Utilizing a menstrual calendar or an app can help individuals keep track of cycle lengths, symptoms, and any irregularities. This information not only serves as a valuable resource for personal awareness but can also aid healthcare providers in assessing menstrual health during medical consultations. By understanding their cycles, young adults can better recognize what is typical for their bodies and when it might be necessary to seek help.

In conclusion, while irregular periods can be concerning, they are often a normal part of the menstrual cycle, especially during the early years. Being informed about the factors that can influence menstrual regularity and keeping track of one's own cycle can empower young adults to take charge of their reproductive health. Open communication with healthcare providers and education about menstrual health are vital components of understanding and managing irregular periods effectively.

Heavy Menstrual Bleeding

Heavy menstrual bleeding, also known as menorrhagia, is a common issue that many young adults may experience during their menstrual cycles. It is characterized by excessive blood loss during menstruation, which can interfere with daily activities and overall quality of life. It is important to understand what constitutes heavy bleeding, as well as the potential causes and symptoms associated with this condition. Generally, heavy menstrual bleeding is defined as losing more than 80 milliliters of blood during each cycle, which can manifest as soaking through one or more sanitary products every hour for several consecutive hours.

Understanding the causes of heavy menstrual bleeding is crucial for effectively managing the condition. Various factors can contribute to menorrhagia, including hormonal imbalances, uterine abnormalities, and certain medical conditions. Hormonal fluctuations, particularly in estrogen and progesterone levels, can lead to an overgrowth of the uterine lining, resulting in heavier periods. Additionally, conditions such as fibroids, polyps, or adenomyosis can physically alter the uterus and increase menstrual flow. Other underlying health issues, such as thyroid disorders, clotting disorders, or pelvic inflammatory disease, may also be responsible for heavier bleeding.

Recognizing the symptoms associated with heavy menstrual bleeding is essential for identifying when to seek medical advice. Symptoms may include prolonged periods lasting more than seven days, the necessity to change sanitary products every hour, and the presence of large blood clots. Some individuals may also experience fatigue, dizziness, or shortness of breath due to blood loss, which can indicate anemia. If any of these symptoms occur consistently, it is advisable to consult a healthcare professional to assess the situation further.

In terms of management, there are several approaches to address heavy menstrual bleeding. Treatment options may vary depending on the underlying cause and severity of the condition. Over-the-counter pain relievers, such as ibuprofen, can help reduce heavy bleeding and alleviate cramps. Hormonal therapies, including birth control pills or hormonal IUDs, can help regulate menstrual cycles and reduce blood flow. In more severe cases, medical procedures such as endometrial ablation or surgery may be recommended. It is crucial to work closely with a healthcare provider to determine the best course of action based on individual circumstances.

Heavy menstrual bleeding can be a challenging experience for many young adults, but it is important to remember that effective management strategies are available. Educating oneself about menstrual health is a vital step in addressing the issue. By understanding the potential causes, recognizing symptoms, and exploring treatment options, individuals can take control of their menstrual health and seek the appropriate support. Remember that heavy menstrual bleeding is not something to suffer in silence; reaching out for help can lead to improved well-being and a more manageable menstrual experience.

Cramps and Pain Management

Cramps, medically known as dysmenorrhea, are a common experience for many individuals during their menstrual cycle. These cramps typically occur in the lower abdomen and can range from mild discomfort to severe pain. The cause of menstrual cramps is often related to the contractions of the uterus as it sheds its lining, driven by hormones called prostaglandins. Higher levels of these hormones can lead to more intense contractions, resulting in increased pain. Understanding the underlying mechanisms of cramps can empower young adults to better manage their symptoms during their periods.

Managing menstrual cramps effectively involves a combination of lifestyle changes and pain relief strategies. Regular exercise is one of the most beneficial practices, as physical activity helps to increase blood flow and reduce the severity of cramps. Activities such as walking, cycling, or yoga can be particularly helpful. Additionally, maintaining a balanced diet that includes anti-inflammatory foods, such as fruits, vegetables, and whole grains, can support overall health and alleviate some menstrual symptoms. Staying hydrated is also crucial, as proper hydration can help reduce bloating and discomfort.

Over-the-counter pain relief medications, such as ibuprofen or naproxen, are commonly used to alleviate menstrual pain. These medications work by reducing the production of prostaglandins, thereby decreasing the intensity of uterine contractions. It is important to follow the recommended dosage and consult with a healthcare professional if symptoms persist or worsen. For those who prefer natural remedies, options such as heat therapy, through heating pads or hot water bottles, can provide significant relief. The warmth helps to relax the muscles of the uterus and improve blood circulation, which can ease cramping.

In some cases, cramps may be a sign of an underlying condition, such as endometriosis or fibroids. These conditions can lead to more severe pain and require specialized medical attention. If cramps are consistently debilitating or accompanied by other symptoms such as heavy bleeding or irregular cycles, it is essential to seek advice from a healthcare provider. They can offer guidance on potential treatments and explore whether further investigation is warranted. Understanding when to seek help is a critical part of managing menstrual health effectively.

Finally, emotional well-being plays a significant role in how individuals experience and cope with menstrual pain. Stress and anxiety can exacerbate feelings of discomfort, so incorporating relaxation techniques such as deep breathing, meditation, or mindfulness can be beneficial. Engaging in supportive communities or discussing experiences with friends can also provide comfort and reduce feelings of isolation. By adopting a holistic approach that combines physical, medical, and emotional strategies, young adults can take charge of their menstrual health and navigate the challenges of cramps more effectively.

Chapter 5: Tracking Your Cycle

Why Track Your Cycle?

Tracking your menstrual cycle is an essential practice that can greatly enhance your understanding of your body and overall health. By keeping a record of your cycle, you can identify patterns and changes that occur over time. This knowledge is empowering, as it allows you to anticipate when your period will start, understand the symptoms you may experience, and recognize any irregularities that could signal a need for medical attention. Being in tune with your cycle helps create a sense of control and minimizes anxiety surrounding menstruation.

One significant reason to track your cycle is to facilitate better communication with healthcare providers. When you have a detailed record of your menstrual cycle, including the length, flow, and symptoms, you can provide your doctor with valuable information during check-ups or when seeking treatment for menstrual-related issues. This information enables healthcare professionals to make informed decisions about your care, whether it involves diagnosing conditions like polycystic ovary syndrome (PCOS) or suggesting appropriate treatments for painful periods.

Additionally, tracking your cycle can help you understand how various factors, such as stress, diet, and exercise, influence your menstrual health. You may notice that certain lifestyle changes impact your cycle's regularity or the severity of symptoms. For instance, increased stress levels might lead to a delayed period, while regular exercise could help alleviate cramps. By observing these relationships, you can make informed choices that promote better menstrual health and overall well-being.

Understanding your cycle can also enhance your reproductive health awareness. Whether you are considering contraception or planning for pregnancy, knowing your cycle can be beneficial. For those looking to conceive, tracking ovulation can help identify the most fertile days, increasing the chance of pregnancy. Conversely, if you wish to avoid pregnancy, understanding your cycle can aid in selecting an effective birth control method that aligns with your body's natural rhythms.

Finally, tracking your menstrual cycle fosters a deeper connection with your body. It encourages mindfulness and self-care, prompting you to take note of your physical and emotional well-being throughout the month. As you become more attuned to your cycle, you may find it easier to recognize changes that warrant attention, leading to a proactive approach to your health. By embracing this practice, you empower yourself to advocate for your health and well-being throughout your life.

Methods of Tracking

Tracking your menstrual cycle is an essential practice for understanding your body and maintaining menstrual health. There are several methods available for tracking your cycle, each offering unique benefits. By becoming familiar with these methods, you can choose the one that best suits your lifestyle and preferences, leading to a greater awareness of your overall health.

One popular method of tracking is using a calendar. This traditional approach involves marking the start and end dates of your period on a physical calendar or planner. By observing your cycle over several months, you can identify patterns in your menstrual flow and predict when your next period is likely to occur. This method is simple, accessible, and requires no special tools, making it ideal for those who prefer a straightforward approach.

Another effective method is the use of mobile applications designed specifically for tracking menstrual cycles. These apps often come equipped with features that allow you to log your period dates, symptoms, mood changes, and any other relevant information. Many of these applications also provide reminders for when your next period is due and some even offer insights into ovulation and fertility. This digital method is convenient and can be easily accessed on-the-go, making it a favored choice for tech-savvy teens.

For those interested in a more detailed understanding of their menstrual health, keeping a journal can be a beneficial method. By writing down daily experiences, including physical symptoms, emotional changes, and lifestyle factors, you can gain deeper insights into how your menstrual cycle affects your life. This method encourages self-reflection and can highlight correlations between your cycle and various aspects of your health, such as stress levels, diet, and exercise routines.

Lastly, some individuals may choose to combine several methods for a comprehensive approach. For instance, using a calendar alongside an app can provide both a visual and digital record of your cycle. Additionally, noting symptoms in a journal can help you understand patterns more clearly. Regardless of the method chosen, tracking your menstrual cycle empowers you to take charge of your health, allowing you to discuss any concerns with healthcare providers more effectively.

Understanding Your Cycle Patterns

Understanding your cycle patterns is essential for managing menstrual health and overall well-being. Each person's menstrual cycle can vary significantly, but most cycles range from 21 to 35 days, with menstruation lasting anywhere from three to seven days. By tracking your cycle, you can gain insights into what is normal for your body, helping you identify any irregularities or changes that may require attention. Familiarizing yourself with your cycle can also empower you to make informed decisions regarding your health.

The menstrual cycle is divided into four main phases: the menstrual phase, the follicular phase, ovulation, and the luteal phase. The menstrual phase begins when the uterus sheds its lining, resulting in bleeding. This phase typically lasts from three to seven days.

Following menstruation, the follicular phase begins, during which the body prepares for ovulation. Hormones such as estrogen rise, stimulating the growth of follicles in the ovaries. Understanding these phases can help you anticipate when your period will start and how you may feel physically and emotionally throughout the month.

Ovulation occurs when a mature egg is released from the ovary, usually around the midpoint of the cycle. This is a crucial time for those who may be trying to conceive, as this is when the chances of pregnancy are highest. Tracking ovulation can also help you recognize your most fertile days, which can be beneficial for understanding your reproductive health. You may notice changes in your body during this time, such as increased cervical mucus or slight changes in basal body temperature, both of which can indicate that ovulation is occurring.

Following ovulation, the luteal phase begins, lasting about 14 days. During this phase, the body prepares for a possible pregnancy. If fertilization does not occur, hormone levels will drop, leading to the onset of menstruation. This phase may come with symptoms associated with premenstrual syndrome (PMS), including mood swings, bloating, and cramps. Being aware of these symptoms can help you manage them effectively and understand that they are a normal part of the cycle for many individuals.

Tracking your cycle can be done through various methods, such as using a calendar, a menstrual tracking app, or simply noting changes in a journal. By recording the start and end dates of your period, any symptoms you experience, and other relevant details, you will create a clearer picture of your cycle. This information can be invaluable for discussions with healthcare providers, allowing for better insights into your menstrual health. Understanding your cycle patterns not only promotes awareness of your body but also fosters a proactive approach to maintaining your reproductive health.

Chapter 6: Nutrition and Menstrual Health

Foods that Support Menstrual Health

Maintaining a healthy diet can significantly impact menstrual health and overall well-being. Certain foods are known to support the body during menstruation by alleviating symptoms such as cramps, bloating, and mood swings. Incorporating these foods into your diet can help you feel more balanced and energized throughout your cycle. This subchapter will explore various food groups that can contribute positively to menstrual health.

Leafy greens, such as spinach, kale, and Swiss chard, are rich in iron and magnesium. These nutrients are crucial for replenishing lost iron during menstruation and may help reduce the severity of cramps. Magnesium can also help relax muscles and ease tension, making it beneficial for those experiencing discomfort. Including a variety of leafy greens in salads, smoothies, or as cooked sides can provide essential nutrients that support your body during your period.

Fruits, particularly those high in antioxidants and vitamins, play a vital role in menstrual health. Berries, oranges, and bananas are excellent choices. Berries are rich in vitamin C, which can help reduce inflammation and support the immune system. Oranges provide hydration and can help combat bloating, while bananas are a great source of potassium, which can alleviate symptoms of water retention and cramping. Incorporating a colorful array of fruits into your diet can not only enhance your mood but also improve your overall health during your cycle.

Whole grains are another essential component of a diet that supports menstrual health. Foods like oats, quinoa, and brown rice are high in fiber, which can help manage blood sugar levels and prevent mood swings often associated with hormonal fluctuations. Whole grains also provide sustained energy, which can be particularly beneficial when fatigue sets in during menstruation. Opting for whole grain options over refined grains can positively impact both physical and mental well-being.

Healthy fats, such as those found in avocados, nuts, and fatty fish, are crucial for hormone regulation and can help reduce inflammation. Omega-3 fatty acids, found in fish like salmon and walnuts, can ease menstrual pain and improve mood. Including sources of healthy fats in your meals can provide essential nutrients that support hormonal balance and overall health. Snacking on nuts or adding avocado to salads can be an easy way to incorporate these beneficial fats into your diet.

Lastly, hydration is a vital yet often overlooked aspect of menstrual health. Drinking plenty of water can help reduce bloating and alleviate headaches that some individuals experience during their cycle. Herbal teas, especially those with anti-inflammatory properties like ginger or chamomile, can provide both hydration and comfort. Staying well-hydrated should be a priority, especially during menstruation, to help maintain energy levels and promote overall wellness. By focusing on these food groups and hydration, you can enhance your menstrual health and navigate your cycle with greater ease.

Supplements and Vitamins

Supplements and vitamins play a significant role in maintaining overall health, especially for those experiencing the physical and emotional changes associated with the menstrual cycle. Understanding which nutrients are beneficial can empower young adults to take control of their menstrual health. Certain vitamins and minerals can alleviate symptoms related to menstruation, enhance energy levels, and support hormonal balance. It is essential to consider these dietary components as part of a holistic approach to menstrual wellness.

Iron is one of the most critical minerals for those who menstruate. During a period, the body loses blood, which can lead to decreased iron levels and potentially result in anemia. Symptoms of iron deficiency may include fatigue, weakness, and irritability. Consuming iron-rich foods, such as red meat, leafy greens, legumes, and fortified cereals, is vital. In some cases, taking an iron supplement may be recommended, especially for individuals with heavy menstrual bleeding or those who follow a vegetarian or vegan diet.

Vitamin B6 is another important nutrient that can help manage premenstrual syndrome (PMS) symptoms. This vitamin supports the production of neurotransmitters that regulate mood and can reduce irritability and emotional fluctuations. Foods rich in B6 include poultry, fish, bananas, and potatoes. For those struggling with severe PMS symptoms, a B6 supplement may be beneficial, but it's crucial to consult a healthcare professional for personalized advice on dosage and safety.

Omega-3 fatty acids are known for their anti-inflammatory properties and can help alleviate menstrual cramps and discomfort. These healthy fats can be found in fatty fish like salmon, flaxseeds, and walnuts. Incorporating omega-3s into the diet may lead to a reduction in period pain and overall menstrual discomfort. Supplements, such as fish oil capsules, are also available for those who may not consume enough omega-3-rich foods.

Lastly, it is essential to approach supplementation with caution. While vitamins and minerals can provide support, they should not replace a balanced diet. Over-supplementation can lead to adverse effects and imbalances. It is advisable for young adults to discuss their specific nutritional needs with a healthcare provider, who can offer guidance on the appropriate use of supplements based on individual health status and lifestyle. Understanding the role of supplements and vitamins in menstrual health can empower teens to make informed decisions and foster a positive relationship with their bodies.

Hydration and Its Importance

Hydration plays a crucial role in maintaining overall health, particularly during menstruation. Water is essential for numerous bodily functions, including digestion, circulation, temperature regulation, and nutrient absorption. During the menstrual cycle, women may experience fluctuations in hormone levels that can lead to various symptoms such as bloating, cramps, and mood swings. Staying properly hydrated can help alleviate some of these symptoms and promote a sense of well-being.

When it comes to menstrual health, hydration can significantly impact how one feels during their cycle. Dehydration can exacerbate symptoms like fatigue and headaches, which are common complaints during menstruation. Drinking enough water helps to flush out toxins and can reduce bloating by improving digestion. Additionally, proper hydration supports overall energy levels, making it easier to manage daily activities and maintain a positive mood.

The amount of water needed can vary based on individual factors such as age, weight, physical activity, and climate. A general guideline is to aim for at least eight 8-ounce glasses of water a day, but some may need more. It is especially important to increase water intake during menstrual periods when the body is losing fluids. Incorporating hydrating foods, such as fruits and vegetables, can also contribute to overall fluid intake and provide essential nutrients.

Many people underestimate the importance of hydration in their daily routines. Staying adequately hydrated can improve focus and cognitive function, which can be beneficial for teens juggling schoolwork, social activities, and other responsibilities. Moreover, hydration can enhance physical performance and recovery, making it an important consideration for those involved in sports or physical activities.

In conclusion, understanding the importance of hydration is vital for menstrual health and overall well-being. By prioritizing fluid intake, young adults can manage menstrual symptoms more effectively and support their bodies during this natural process. Developing healthy hydration habits not only benefits menstrual health but also lays the foundation for a lifetime of wellness.

Chapter 7: Emotional Well-being and Menstruation

Mood Swings and Hormonal Changes

Hormonal changes throughout the menstrual cycle can significantly influence mood and emotional well-being. Understanding these fluctuations is essential for young adults as they navigate their teenage years. The menstrual cycle is divided into phases, each characterized by varying levels of hormones like estrogen and progesterone. These hormonal shifts can impact neurotransmitters in the brain, which are responsible for regulating mood. As estrogen levels rise during the follicular phase, individuals may feel more energetic and positive. Conversely, as the cycle progresses and progesterone levels increase during the luteal phase, some may experience heightened emotions or irritability.

The premenstrual phase, often referred to as premenstrual syndrome (PMS), can bring about notable mood swings for many individuals. Symptoms of PMS can include anxiety, depression, and irritability, which can be attributed to the drop in estrogen and the rise in progesterone. These emotional changes can affect daily life, including relationships, academic performance, and overall quality of life. Recognizing that these feelings are often linked to hormonal changes can help individuals approach them with more understanding and compassion towards themselves.

Some young adults may experience more severe emotional changes, known as premenstrual dysphoric disorder (PMDD). PMDD is a more intense form of PMS that can significantly disrupt daily life. Symptoms may include severe mood swings, irritability, and feelings of hopelessness. It is important for those who suspect they may be experiencing PMDD to seek guidance from a healthcare professional. Understanding the difference between PMS and PMDD can empower young adults to communicate their experiences and seek appropriate support.

Lifestyle choices can also have a profound impact on mood during the menstrual cycle. Regular physical activity, a balanced diet, and adequate sleep can help mitigate some of the mood swings associated with hormonal changes. Engaging in activities that promote relaxation, such as yoga or meditation, can also be beneficial. These practices can help balance hormones and improve overall emotional health, making it easier to cope with the ups and downs of the menstrual cycle.

In conclusion, recognizing the connection between hormonal changes and mood swings is vital for young adults as they learn to manage their menstrual health. By understanding the phases of the cycle and their effects on emotional well-being, individuals can better navigate their feelings and respond to them in constructive ways. With this knowledge, young adults can cultivate a more positive relationship with their bodies and emotions, leading to greater overall wellness during their menstrual cycles.

Coping Mechanisms

Coping mechanisms are essential tools that help individuals manage the physical and emotional symptoms associated with the menstrual cycle. Understanding these mechanisms can empower young adults to navigate their menstrual health more effectively. Different coping strategies can be employed to alleviate discomfort, reduce stress, and promote overall well-being. By identifying what works best for oneself, it becomes easier to face the challenges that may arise during different phases of the cycle.

One common coping mechanism is engaging in physical activity. Exercise can significantly improve mood and reduce menstrual pain. Activities such as walking, yoga, or dancing can release endorphins, the body's natural painkillers, and mood elevators. Incorporating regular physical activity into one's routine not only helps manage symptoms but also encourages a healthier lifestyle overall. Finding enjoyable activities can transform exercise from a chore into a pleasurable part of daily life.

Another effective coping strategy involves dietary adjustments. Nutrition plays a crucial role in menstrual health, and certain foods can help alleviate symptoms. For instance, incorporating more fruits, vegetables, whole grains, and lean proteins can provide the body with essential nutrients. Additionally, staying hydrated and reducing caffeine and sugary foods can minimize bloating and irritability. Keeping a food diary can help identify which foods positively or negatively affect one's cycle, allowing for better choices in the future.

Mindfulness and relaxation techniques are also valuable coping mechanisms. Practices such as meditation, deep breathing exercises, and journaling can help manage stress and anxiety that may accompany menstrual symptoms. Taking time to relax and reflect can create a sense of control and calmness. Establishing a calming routine during menstrual phases can make a significant difference, providing a mental space to process emotions and physical sensations.

Finally, seeking support from friends, family, or support groups can be an important aspect of coping with menstrual health. Sharing experiences and feelings can foster connection and understanding. It is crucial to create an environment where discussing menstrual health is normalized, as this can significantly reduce feelings of isolation or shame. Engaging with others who understand the challenges can provide reassurance and practical advice, making the journey through the menstrual cycle more manageable and less daunting.

Seeking Support

Seeking support during your menstrual cycle is a crucial aspect of understanding and managing your menstrual health. Many young adults may feel isolated or unsure about their experiences, but it is important to recognize that seeking help is a common and healthy response. Support can come from various sources, including friends, family, educators, and healthcare professionals. By reaching out, you can gain valuable insights, share experiences, and find comfort in knowing that you are not alone in navigating the complexities of your menstrual health.

One of the most accessible sources of support is your circle of friends. Friends who are also experiencing their cycles can be particularly understanding and relatable. Sharing your experiences with them can foster a sense of camaraderie and provide emotional relief. It can also be an opportunity to discuss tips and tricks for managing symptoms like cramps or mood swings. Creating a safe space to talk openly about periods can help normalize the conversation and reduce any stigma associated with menstruation.

Family members, particularly female relatives, can also be a great source of support. They may have valuable experiences and wisdom to share about their own menstrual journeys. Talking to a parent or sibling can offer insights into managing menstrual symptoms or navigating the emotional ups and downs that can accompany your cycle. Moreover, discussing menstruation with family can strengthen bonds and encourage a more open dialogue about health and wellness within the household.

Educators and school health professionals can play a pivotal role in providing support and information. Schools often have resources available, such as health education classes or counseling services, where you can learn more about menstrual health and ask questions in a safe environment. These professionals can help clarify any misconceptions and provide accurate information about your body and menstrual cycle. Don't hesitate to approach a trusted teacher or school nurse if you need guidance or support.

Lastly, healthcare professionals should not be overlooked when seeking support. If you have concerns about your menstrual health or experience severe symptoms, scheduling an appointment with a doctor or gynecologist can be beneficial. They can offer personalized advice, diagnose any potential issues, and discuss treatment options. Understanding your menstrual health is an essential part of overall well-being, and healthcare providers are there to help you navigate this journey. Remember, seeking support is a sign of strength and a vital step in taking charge of your menstrual health.

Chapter 8: Myths and Misconceptions

Common Myths About Menstruation

Menstruation is often surrounded by a cloud of myths and misconceptions that can lead to confusion and anxiety among young adults. One of the most pervasive myths is that menstruation is inherently dirty or shameful. This stigma can create feelings of embarrassment and secrecy, making it difficult for individuals to discuss their menstrual health openly. In reality, menstruation is a natural biological process that signifies a healthy reproductive system. Understanding this can help normalize the conversation around periods and empower individuals to embrace their menstrual health with confidence.

Another common misconception is that menstruation is always painful. While many individuals experience discomfort or cramps, this is not the case for everyone. Each person's experience with menstruation is unique, and symptoms can vary widely. Some may have mild or no symptoms at all, while others may experience severe pain known as dysmenorrhea. It is important to recognize that experiencing pain is not a universal truth of menstruation, and those who do experience discomfort should seek advice and treatment options from healthcare professionals.

Many young adults also believe that engaging in physical activities or sports during menstruation is harmful. This myth can discourage individuals from maintaining an active lifestyle during their periods. In fact, exercise can be beneficial during menstruation, as it can reduce cramps, improve mood, and boost energy levels. Understanding that physical activity is not only safe but can actually enhance well-being during menstruation allows individuals to continue their routines without fear or hesitation.

Another misconception is that menstruation should last a specific number of days. While many people experience a menstrual cycle that lasts between three to seven days, variations are completely normal. Factors such as age, hormonal changes, and stress can influence cycle length. Young adults should be educated about what constitutes a typical cycle for them while understanding that variations are part of the natural process. This knowledge can help alleviate anxiety and encourage individuals to track their cycles for better health management.

Lastly, there is a myth that menstrual blood is toxic or harmful. This misconception can perpetuate fear and misunderstanding about menstruation. Menstrual blood is simply a combination of blood, uterine lining, and vaginal secretions, and it is not harmful. Understanding this fact can help dismantle the stigma surrounding menstruation and encourage a healthier dialogue about menstrual health. By debunking these common myths, young adults can foster a more supportive and informed environment regarding menstruation and overall reproductive health.

Debunking Misconceptions

Misconceptions about menstruation are widespread and can lead to confusion and anxiety among young adults. One common myth is that menstruation is a dirty or shameful process. This belief often stems from cultural taboos and misinformation. In reality, menstruation is a natural biological function that is essential for reproductive health. Understanding that menstruation is a normal part of life can help normalize the conversation around it, allowing for healthier discussions and attitudes toward this important aspect of health.

Another misconception is that menstruation only affects girls and women. While it is true that only individuals with a uterus and ovaries experience menstrual cycles, the impact of menstruation extends to everyone. Menstruation can affect relationships, social activities, and mental health. Young men and non-binary individuals should also be educated about menstruation to foster an inclusive environment. When everyone understands menstruation, it can help break down stigma and create a supportive community for those who experience it.

Some young adults believe that they cannot engage in physical activities, such as sports or swimming, during their periods. This is simply untrue. Many people continue their regular activities while menstruating. With the right products, such as pads, tampons, or menstrual cups, individuals can comfortably participate in any activity. It's important to listen to one's body and adapt as needed, but there is no reason to avoid physical activities simply because of menstruation.

Another area of misunderstanding is the belief that menstrual cycles are always regular and predictable. While some individuals do have regular cycles, others may experience irregularities due to various factors, including stress, diet, or underlying health conditions. Recognizing that menstrual cycles can vary greatly from person to person can help alleviate concerns about one's health. Tracking cycles can empower individuals to better understand their bodies and identify any patterns or changes that may require medical attention.

Lastly, there is a misconception that menstrual pain, known as dysmenorrhea, is something that all individuals must simply endure. While some discomfort is common, severe pain is not normal and can be a sign of underlying issues such as endometriosis or fibroids. It is essential for young adults to understand that they should seek help if they experience debilitating pain. Open discussions about menstrual pain can lead to better treatment options and improved quality of life for those affected. By debunking these misconceptions, we can foster a more informed and supportive environment for all individuals experiencing menstruation.

Chapter 9: Period Products

Overview of Menstrual Products

Menstrual products are essential tools that help individuals manage their menstrual flow effectively. Understanding the various options available can empower young adults to make informed choices that suit their lifestyles and preferences. The most common menstrual products include pads, tampons, menstrual cups, and period underwear, each with its unique features and benefits. Choosing the right product can enhance comfort, convenience, and confidence during menstruation.

Sanitary pads are one of the oldest and most widely used menstrual products. They come in various sizes and absorbencies, catering to different flow levels. Pads are simple to use; they adhere to the inside of underwear and absorb menstrual blood as it flows. Some pads are designed for overnight use, featuring extra absorbency and longer lengths to prevent leaks while sleeping. Additionally, pads are available in both disposable and reusable options, allowing users to select based on their preferences and environmental considerations.

Tampons are another popular choice for menstrual management. They are made of absorbent material and are inserted into the vaginal canal to absorb menstrual fluid internally. This allows for greater freedom of movement and the ability to engage in activities such as swimming or sports without the worry of leaks. Tampons come in various absorbency levels, which are particularly important to consider during the first few days of menstruation when flow tends to be heavier. It is vital for users to follow guidelines on safe usage to minimize risks, such as Toxic Shock Syndrome.

Menstrual cups have gained popularity in recent years due to their eco-friendliness and cost-effectiveness. These flexible cups are made from silicone or rubber and are inserted into the vaginal canal to collect menstrual fluid. Unlike pads and tampons, menstrual cups can be reused for several years with proper care, making them a sustainable option. They come in different sizes and shapes, allowing users to choose one that fits their anatomy comfortably. While there may be a learning curve for first-time users, many find menstrual cups to be a convenient and reliable option once they become familiar with them.

Period underwear is an innovative solution that combines comfort and protection. Designed to look and feel like regular underwear, these garments have built-in absorbent layers that can hold menstrual fluid, making them suitable for light to moderate flow days. They can be worn alone or as a backup to other menstrual products. Available in various styles and absorbency levels, period underwear offers a discreet and comfortable alternative. As menstrual health continues to evolve, understanding these products can help young adults navigate their options and find the best fit for their needs, promoting a positive experience during their menstrual cycle.

Choosing the Right Product for You

Choosing the right menstrual product is an important aspect of menstrual health. With a variety of options available, it can be overwhelming to determine which product best suits your individual needs. Factors such as comfort, absorbency, convenience, and environmental impact can influence your choice. Understanding these aspects will help you make an informed decision that aligns with your lifestyle and preferences.

One of the most common options is disposable pads. They come in various sizes and absorbencies, making them suitable for different flow levels. Pads are easy to use and widely available, which adds to their convenience. However, some may find them bulky or uncomfortable. It's essential to try different brands to find the right fit for your body and comfort level. Additionally, consider how often you will need to change them throughout the day, as this can impact your overall comfort and hygiene.

Tampons are another popular choice and can be more discreet than pads. They are inserted into the vagina, which can make them feel less noticeable during physical activities. Tampons also come in various absorbency levels, allowing you to choose one that fits your flow. However, it's crucial to understand how to use them properly to avoid risks such as Toxic Shock Syndrome (TSS). Familiarizing yourself with the instructions and following hygiene practices will ensure a safe experience with tampons.

For those interested in more sustainable options, menstrual cups and reusable cloth pads are becoming increasingly popular. Menstrual cups are flexible cups made of silicone or rubber that collect menstrual fluid. They can be worn for up to 12 hours, depending on your flow, and are reusable for several years. This option can significantly reduce waste and save money over time. Reusable cloth pads, on the other hand, offer comfort and can be customized in terms of design and absorbency. They do require more maintenance, as they need to be washed and dried, but many users find them to be a more environmentally friendly choice.

Ultimately, the right product for you will depend on your personal preferences and lifestyle. It's essential to consider factors such as your activity level, flow, and any sensitivities or allergies you may have. Experimenting with different products can help you discover what feels best for your body. Remember that it's perfectly normal to switch between products based on your needs, and there's no one-size-fits-all solution. Taking the time to choose the right menstrual product will enhance your comfort and confidence during your cycle.

Eco-Friendly Options

When considering menstrual health, eco-friendly options not only contribute to personal well-being but also promote environmental sustainability. The menstrual products traditionally advertised often come with substantial ecological footprints, primarily due to their packaging and the materials used in their production. By opting for more sustainable alternatives, individuals can minimize waste and reduce their impact on the planet while managing their menstrual health effectively.

One popular eco-friendly option is reusable menstrual cups. Made from medical-grade silicone, rubber, or latex, menstrual cups can be used for several years, significantly reducing the amount of waste generated from disposable products. They are designed to collect menstrual fluid rather than absorb it, which can lead to a lower risk of irritation and infections. Additionally, menstrual cups can hold more fluid than most pads or tampons, allowing for longer wear time before needing to be emptied. This combination of longevity and practicality makes them a compelling choice for those looking to embrace sustainability.

Cloth menstrual pads are another excellent eco-friendly alternative. These pads are made from natural materials, such as cotton or bamboo, and can be washed and reused. By choosing cloth pads, individuals can avoid the synthetic materials found in many disposable options, which can take hundreds of years to decompose. Cloth pads come in various sizes and absorbencies, allowing users to tailor their menstrual care to their specific needs. Furthermore, many brands offer stylish designs and patterns, making them an appealing choice for those who prioritize both functionality and aesthetics.

Period underwear has also gained popularity as a sustainable option. These specially designed garments incorporate absorbent layers that can hold menstrual flow, providing a comfortable and discreet alternative to traditional products. Depending on the brand and style, period underwear can be worn alone or as backup protection alongside other menstrual products. They are machine washable and can last for several years, making them an economical and environmentally-friendly choice. By incorporating period underwear into their menstrual health routine, individuals can significantly reduce the waste associated with disposables.

Finally, it is essential to consider the overall impact of menstrual product choices on the environment. Educating oneself about the ingredients and manufacturing processes of menstrual products can help in making informed decisions. Many eco-friendly options not only reduce waste but also support ethical labor practices and sustainable sourcing. By choosing products that align with personal values regarding health and the environment, individuals can advocate for a more sustainable future while taking care of their menstrual health.

Chapter 10: When to Seek Medical Advice

Signs of Potential Issues

Recognizing the signs of potential issues related to menstrual health is crucial for young adults. Understanding what is considered normal and what may indicate a problem can help individuals take proactive steps in managing their health. There are various physical and emotional signals that may suggest an underlying issue with the menstrual cycle. Being aware of these signs can empower teens to seek help when necessary and foster a better understanding of their bodies.

One common sign of potential issues is irregular periods. While it is normal for cycles to vary during the first few years after menstruation begins, consistently irregular cycles may warrant attention. This can include periods that are excessively long, short, or unpredictable. Irregular cycles can be caused by several factors, including hormonal imbalances, stress, weight changes, or underlying health conditions. Tracking menstrual cycles using a calendar or an app can help identify patterns and variations that may signal a need for further evaluation.

Another indicator of potential menstrual health issues is severe pain during menstruation, known as dysmenorrhea. While some discomfort is common, intense pain that interferes with daily activities may suggest conditions such as endometriosis or fibroids. It is important to differentiate between typical menstrual cramps and pain that is debilitating. If over-the-counter pain relievers do not provide relief, or if pain persists outside of menstruation, consulting a healthcare provider is advisable.

Changes in menstrual flow can also indicate potential issues. A significant increase or decrease in bleeding, or the passing of large clots, can signal hormonal imbalances or other medical conditions. Heavy bleeding, known as menorrhagia, can lead to anemia and other health concerns if left unaddressed. Conversely, very light periods may be a sign of conditions like polycystic ovary syndrome (PCOS) or other hormonal disorders. Monitoring menstrual flow and discussing any concerns with a healthcare professional is essential for maintaining menstrual health.

Emotional and psychological changes associated with the menstrual cycle can also provide insight into potential problems. Many individuals experience mood swings, irritability, or anxiety as part of premenstrual syndrome (PMS). However, if these symptoms are severe or debilitating, they may be indicative of premenstrual dysphoric disorder (PMDD) or other mental health concerns. It is important to recognize when emotional symptoms interfere with daily life and to seek support from a trusted adult or mental health professional if necessary. Understanding these signs can lead to better menstrual health management and overall well-being.

Talking to a Healthcare Professional

Talking to a healthcare professional about menstrual health is an important step in understanding your body and addressing any concerns you may have. Whether you are experiencing irregular periods, severe cramps, or other symptoms, healthcare providers are trained to help guide you through these issues. It is essential to approach these conversations with an open mind and a willingness to share your experiences honestly. This not only helps your provider understand your situation better but also fosters a trusting relationship, which is crucial for effective healthcare.

Before your appointment, it can be helpful to prepare a list of questions or concerns you wish to discuss. This might include inquiries about what is considered a normal menstrual cycle, the impact of stress on your periods, or the various options available for managing painful symptoms. Additionally, keeping track of your menstrual cycle using a journal or an app can provide valuable insights to share with your healthcare professional. This information can assist them in making an accurate assessment and recommendation tailored to your needs.

During your visit, feel free to express your feelings and thoughts about your menstrual health. Discuss any symptoms you are experiencing, such as mood swings, bloating, or changes in your cycle. Remember that no concern is too small or insignificant; healthcare professionals are accustomed to discussing a wide range of menstrual-related issues. If you feel embarrassed or uncomfortable, remind yourself that these professionals are there to help you and have likely heard similar concerns from other patients.

It's also important to understand the various options available for managing menstrual health. Your healthcare provider might suggest lifestyle changes, over-the-counter medications, or even hormonal treatments, depending on your specific situation. Ask questions about the benefits and potential side effects of any proposed treatments. Understanding these options empowers you to make informed decisions about your health, ensuring that you choose the best path forward for your body.

Finally, remember that you have the right to seek a second opinion if you feel your concerns are not being adequately addressed. Finding a healthcare professional you feel comfortable with is essential for ongoing health discussions. Whether it's a pediatrician, gynecologist, or family doctor, make sure you feel heard and respected. Your menstrual health is an integral part of your overall well-being, and having a supportive healthcare provider can make all the difference in navigating this important aspect of your life.

Chapter 11: Empowering Yourself and Others

Advocacy for Menstrual Health

Advocacy for menstrual health is crucial for fostering a supportive environment where young people can learn about and manage their cycles effectively. Menstrual health encompasses not only the physiological aspects of menstruation but also the social, emotional, and educational factors that influence how individuals experience their periods. As a young adult, understanding the importance of advocacy in this area can empower you to take action, support your peers, and promote a culture of openness and education surrounding menstrual health.

One significant aspect of menstrual health advocacy is education. Many young people lack comprehensive knowledge about menstruation, often relying on outdated myths or limited information. By advocating for accurate and inclusive menstrual health education in schools and communities, you can help ensure that everyone has access to the information they need. This includes not only the biological processes involved but also discussions about menstrual hygiene, the emotional impacts of menstruation, and the variety of experiences individuals may have. Education fosters understanding and reduces stigma, allowing for more informed conversations about menstrual health.

Another critical area for advocacy is access to menstrual products. Many individuals face barriers to obtaining necessary supplies due to financial constraints, lack of availability, or inadequate support from their environments. Promoting initiatives that provide free or affordable menstrual products in schools and community centers can help alleviate this issue. Additionally, advocating for policies that ensure menstrual products are included in basic health care and emergency assistance programs is essential. Ensuring that everyone has access to the products they need is a fundamental aspect of menstrual health.

Mental health and emotional well-being are often overlooked in discussions about menstrual health, yet they are vital components of the overall experience. Advocacy efforts should include raising awareness of the emotional challenges that may accompany menstruation, such as premenstrual syndrome (PMS) and other menstrual-related disorders. By encouraging open dialogue about these issues, you can help reduce the stigma and isolation that many face. Mental health resources and support systems must be integrated into menstrual health discussions to provide young adults with the tools they need to manage their emotional well-being effectively.

Finally, intersectionality plays a significant role in menstrual health advocacy. Recognizing that different backgrounds, cultures, and experiences shape how individuals perceive and manage their menstrual health is essential. Advocacy should aim to be inclusive, addressing the unique needs of marginalized groups who may face additional challenges related to menstruation. By promoting diverse voices and experiences in menstrual health discussions, you can help create a more equitable landscape where all individuals feel represented and supported in their menstrual health journeys.

Sharing Knowledge with Peers

Sharing knowledge about menstrual health with peers is an essential aspect of fostering a supportive environment for young adults. When individuals openly discuss their experiences and understanding of menstrual cycles, they not only empower themselves but also create a culture of understanding and respect among their peers. This sharing can take place in various settings, whether in classrooms, social gatherings, or online platforms, and plays a crucial role in breaking down stigmas associated with menstruation.

One effective way to share knowledge is through organized discussion groups or workshops. These gatherings provide a safe space for individuals to ask questions, share personal stories, and learn from one another. Such interactions can help dispel myths and misconceptions surrounding menstruation, promoting accurate information. By inviting healthcare professionals or educators to facilitate these sessions, participants can gain access to reliable resources and expert insights, which can enhance their understanding of menstrual health.

Additionally, leveraging social media platforms can significantly amplify the reach of menstrual health education. Young adults are already engaging with various online communities, making it a prime avenue for sharing knowledge. By creating informative content such as blog posts, videos, or infographics, individuals can educate their peers in an engaging and relatable manner. This digital approach not only normalizes conversations around menstruation but also allows for the sharing of personal journeys, fostering a sense of solidarity among those navigating similar experiences.

Peer-led initiatives, such as school clubs focused on health education, can also be instrumental in promoting awareness. These clubs can organize events, distribute educational materials, and create campaigns that encourage open dialogue about menstrual health. By taking the initiative to lead these discussions, young adults can inspire others to share their knowledge and experiences, contributing to a more informed and compassionate community. Furthermore, these initiatives can help develop leadership skills and confidence in participants, empowering them to advocate for menstrual health education.

Ultimately, sharing knowledge with peers is about creating an informed and supportive network. As young adults engage in conversations about menstrual health, they not only enhance their own understanding but also play a crucial role in educating others. By fostering an environment where menstruation is openly discussed, stigmas can be challenged, and individuals can feel more comfortable and confident in their bodies. This collective effort is vital for advancing menstrual health education and ensuring that all young people have access to the information they need to navigate their cycles with confidence and care.

Building a Supportive Community

Building a supportive community around menstrual health can significantly enhance the experience of young adults navigating this essential aspect of life. A supportive community provides a safe space for individuals to share their experiences, seek advice, and learn from one another. This sense of belonging can help alleviate feelings of isolation and confusion that often accompany the onset of menstruation. Creating such a community begins with fostering open dialogue about menstrual health, breaking down the stigma that often surrounds these conversations.

One of the first steps in building a supportive community is encouraging open discussions about menstruation among peers. This can be initiated in various settings, such as schools, community centers, or even online platforms. By creating forums where young adults feel comfortable sharing their experiences, questions, and concerns, we can normalize conversations about menstrual health. These discussions can also help dispel myths and misconceptions, allowing individuals to gain accurate information that empowers them to manage their menstrual health more effectively.

In addition to peer-to-peer discussions, involving educators and healthcare professionals can enrich the community. Workshops and seminars led by knowledgeable individuals can provide valuable insights into menstrual health, including topics like cycle tracking, managing symptoms, and understanding the hormonal changes that occur during the menstrual cycle. By integrating expert advice into community activities, young adults can access reliable information that can aid them in making informed decisions about their health.

Supportive communities can also extend beyond discussions and educational opportunities. Peer support groups can be established where individuals can share their experiences and coping strategies. These groups can serve as a foundation for building friendships and connections among individuals who share similar experiences. Additionally, creating online platforms or social media groups can facilitate ongoing support, allowing members to connect, share resources, and provide encouragement to one another, regardless of geographic location.

Ultimately, building a supportive community for menstrual health is about creating an environment where young adults feel empowered to understand and embrace their bodies. By fostering open dialogue, integrating expert knowledge, and encouraging peer support, we can cultivate a culture that values menstrual health and wellness. This community not only benefits individuals as they navigate their cycles but also contributes to broader societal change by challenging stigma and promoting awareness about menstrual health.

Chapter 12: Resources for Further Learning

Books and Articles

Books and articles play a crucial role in providing information about menstrual health, especially for young adults who are navigating their own cycles for the first time. These resources offer a wealth of knowledge, ranging from the biological aspects of menstruation to the emotional and social implications that come with it. Understanding menstrual health is not just about knowing when to expect your period; it encompasses recognizing symptoms, managing discomfort, and understanding the impact of hormonal changes on mood and behavior.

Several books focus specifically on menstrual health, catering to the unique needs of young adults. Titles such as "The Period Repair Manual" by Lara Briden and "Cycle Syncing" by Alisa Vitti provide insights into the menstrual cycle's phases and how they affect physical and emotional well-being. These authors emphasize the importance of recognizing individual patterns and how lifestyle choices, like diet and exercise, can influence menstrual health. Such resources encourage readers to take an active role in their health and provide practical tips for managing their cycles effectively.

In addition to books, numerous articles in magazines, blogs, and scientific journals address menstrual health topics relevant to teens and young adults. Websites like Planned Parenthood and the American College of Obstetricians and Gynecologists offer articles that cover everything from the basics of menstruation to more complex issues like hormonal birth control and menstrual disorders. These articles are often written in an accessible language, making it easy for readers to understand and apply the information to their lives.

Furthermore, the advent of online platforms has led to an increase in accessible menstrual health education. Many blogs and social media accounts are dedicated to demystifying menstruation and breaking the stigma surrounding it. Influencers and health professionals often share their personal experiences and expert advice, creating a community where young adults can learn and ask questions in a safe environment. This peer-to-peer sharing of knowledge can be especially valuable for those who may feel uncomfortable discussing menstrual health in traditional settings.

It is essential for young adults to engage with a variety of these resources to build a comprehensive understanding of their menstrual health. By reading books and articles, they can obtain factual information, dispel myths, and learn about the diverse experiences of others. This knowledge empowers them to make informed decisions regarding their bodies and health, paving the way for a more positive relationship with their menstrual cycles and overall well-being.

Online Platforms and Communities

Online platforms and communities have become essential resources for young adults seeking information and support regarding menstrual health. With the rise of social media and various websites dedicated to health education, teens can access a wealth of knowledge about their menstrual cycles. These platforms not only provide factual information but also create safe spaces where young adults can share their experiences, ask questions, and connect with others who may be going through similar situations. This sense of community can be particularly valuable in an area often surrounded by stigma and misinformation.

Social media platforms such as Instagram, TikTok, and Twitter have emerged as popular venues for menstrual health discussions. Influencers, health educators, and organizations use these channels to disseminate information in engaging and relatable ways. Content often includes tips for tracking cycles, advice on managing symptoms, and discussions about the emotional aspects of menstruation. The creative formats—such as infographics, videos, and live Q&A sessions—make complex topics more accessible and enjoyable for young audiences. This approach helps normalize conversations around menstruation, encouraging more teens to seek the information they need.

In addition to social media, dedicated online communities and forums offer a more focused environment for discussions about menstrual health. Websites such as Reddit and health-focused forums allow users to ask questions and share personal stories anonymously. This anonymity can empower young adults to discuss sensitive topics they might hesitate to bring up in person, such as irregular cycles, severe cramps, or the emotional impact of menstruation. These platforms foster a sense of belonging and support, enabling users to learn from one another's experiences and coping strategies.

Educational websites and blogs run by healthcare professionals also play a crucial role in providing accurate information. These resources often include articles, videos, and downloadable guides that cover a wide range of topics related to menstrual health, from understanding the menstrual cycle to recognizing signs of conditions like PCOS or endometriosis. Young adults can rely on these reputable sources to clarify misconceptions and learn about their bodies, ensuring they receive reliable information rather than unverified advice from less credible sources.

While online platforms and communities offer valuable resources, it is essential for young adults to approach these spaces critically. Not all information shared online is accurate, and some discussions may perpetuate myths or stigma. It is important for teens to cross-reference information with reputable sources, such as healthcare providers or established health organizations. By doing so, they can empower themselves with knowledge and make informed decisions about their menstrual health, all while benefiting from the supportive networks that online communities provide.

Health Organizations and Hotlines

Health organizations and hotlines play a crucial role in providing accurate information, support, and resources related to menstrual health. For teens navigating the complexities of their cycles, these resources can be invaluable. Various national and local organizations focus on menstrual health, offering educational materials, advocacy, and community support. Understanding how to access these resources can empower young adults to take charge of their menstrual health and make informed decisions.

One prominent organization dedicated to menstrual health is Planned Parenthood. They offer a wealth of information on reproductive health, including detailed explanations of the menstrual cycle, common issues such as cramps and irregular periods, and advice on managing symptoms. Planned Parenthood also provides access to health services, including consultations and treatments for menstrual-related concerns. Their website features resources tailored for teens, ensuring that young adults have the knowledge they need to understand their bodies.

Another valuable resource is the American College of Obstetricians and Gynecologists (ACOG). ACOG focuses on education and advocacy related to women's health, including menstrual health. Their website includes articles, FAQs, and downloadable resources specifically geared toward adolescents. Additionally, ACOG promotes the importance of regular gynecological check-ups, encouraging teens to discuss menstrual health openly with their healthcare providers. This proactive approach can help young adults feel more comfortable in managing their menstrual health.

Hotlines also serve as an essential resource for teens seeking immediate support or guidance. Organizations like the National Women's Health Network provide toll-free numbers where young adults can speak with trained professionals about their menstrual health questions or concerns. These hotlines offer confidential support, helping teens navigate issues such as menstrual irregularities, pain management, and emotional well-being related to their cycles. Accessing a hotline can provide reassurance and information in moments of confusion or distress.

In addition to these national organizations, many local health departments and community centers offer services and resources tailored to young adults. These organizations often conduct workshops, provide educational materials, and create safe spaces for teens to discuss their experiences. By connecting with local resources, young adults can find support that is both accessible and relevant to their unique needs. Understanding the available health organizations and hotlines can empower teens to take control of their menstrual health and foster a sense of community in their journey.